Saliva Enzymes: The Important Function Of Saliva Enzymes And How To Improve Your Health Through Understanding

Disclaimer and Terms of Use: Effort has been made to ensure that the information in this book is accurate and complete, however, the author and the publisher do not warrant the accuracy of the information, text and graphics contained within the book due to the rapidly changing nature of science, research, known and unknown facts and internet. The Author and the publisher do not hold any responsibility for errors, omissions or contrary interpretation of the subject matter herein. This book is presented solely for motivational and informational purposes only.

Table of Contents

Introduction

Saliva is produced by all human individual, including all other animals. It contains water in much of its substance and somewhat frothy in nature. Produced in the mouth, saliva is formed by salivary glands present in our body. Digestion of our food is primarily dependent on mixing of saliva with our food in the mouth itself. Our body produces saliva when the food reaches inside the mouth and at the time when chewing process is taking place. Saliva serves as lubricants of the food. In that way saliva produced by salivary gland moistens the food and creates a bolus within mouth. This process makes the swallowing of the bolus very easy in order to reach to the stomach for second phase of digestion.

Actually many people has misconception that digestion of food occurs in the stomach but it actually starts in the mouth and it is the primary process that makes digestion possible. Saliva also protects from desiccation to oral surfaces.

Content Of Saliva

Other than 98% of the water saliva contains other substances which is as follows

- Electrolytes

- Mucus

- Glycoprotein

- Few antibacterial compounds like IgA and Lysozyme

- And many other enzymes

The amount of water in saliva may vary from 97%to 99.5%. On an average it contains 98%.

Saliva Enzymes

Saliva enzymes are mainly the aiding agents in assisting the body in various digestive and metabolic processes. It is one type of catalyst substance. These protein structure enzymes are mainly plays a role in increasing the speed of metabolic activities and decreases the time taken to digest the food for better digestion.

Types Of Salivary Enzymes

There are number of saliva enzymes formed in our mouth by salivary gland and each enzyme has vital role to play. Salivary enzymes presented in the mouth are mentioned below

- Ptyalin

- Amylase

- Betaine

- Bromelain

Structural Mechanism Of Salivary Enzymes

Enzymes are nothing but globular proteins. Enzymes contain mainly 62 amino acids. Saliva enzymes has mostly a three dimensional structure.

- The structure and size of the enzymes are much larger than any substances they are reacting on for catalyst activities.

- The site which is important to carry out enzyme reaction with the substance is called as "active sites"

- There is a part of enzyme which is able to bind the cofactors. This cofactor is very essential components in helps in catalysing process.

- Apart from cofactors, these enzymes also has place to bind molecules not the big ones but small. These small molecules can be from direct or indirect processes. Due to this binding process the speed of the enzymes can increase or decrease.

- As it is known that saliva enzymes are sequence of amino acids which has its own unique properties. Based on this property the function of each saliva enzymes varies and there amino acid sometimes binds together in groups creating a protein complex.

Unique Specificity

Each of the saliva Enzymes has a very specific role to play and it is in their very nature. They react to only specific activities and not by any other activities. For example to break down starch and converts it into small and simple sugar molecule is the function of amylase, this function cannot be processed or initiated by any other enzymes even though there are many enzymes that are present in the saliva.

Working Model

Saliva enzymes have their own specific shape and structure. When the enzymes are processing inside the mouth they bind with the substrates. Substrate fits exactly on the enzymes and it makes the way clear for the processes. It is commonly being referred as lock and key model. These molecules can change the shape in order to adjust to the active sites to bind. And the active site of the enzyme also changes its shape to bind the substrate molecules.

Action Mechanisms And Important Properties

Saliva enzymes works on the several functional mechanisms that are vital in order to complete the activities, some specific mechanisms are as of following

- Maintaining the shape of enzyme is very important in order to carry our reactions. If the shape of this enzyme get disrupted then it losses the ability to complete the function.

- Temperature has positive accelerating effect on the activities of enzymes. Temperature commonly speeds up the process to develop the product at faster rates. In case of extreme temperature saliva enzymes can lose its original properties and becomes denatured. Although there is some saliva enzyme which works at their best in low temperature.

- If the digestive or any other process can't be completed in one step then it may provide with an alternative pathway.

- It reduces the energy wastage in transition. When saliva enzymes bind with the substances or molecules it goes into transition state in order to reach to the ultimate state.

Functions Of The Salivary Enzymes

The salivary gland secretes many types of mouth enzymes to aid in initiating the first process of digestion. Lysozyme is one of the enzymes secreted by salivary gland which has natural antibacterial action. It provides protection to mouth from harmful bacteria.

Salivary enzymes serve with the variety of functions to aid the proper functioning of our body and other crucial bodily functions

1. **Ptyalin:** It serves as a catalyst in converting starch into simple sugar components

2. **Amylase:** It almost serves the same function as the ptyalin but it converts the sugar into simpler format. This breakdown of starch into simple molecules of sugar is being absorbed in the blood, increasing the blood glucose level. To maintain the proper health maintaining of blood glucose level is very important. The amount of food digested and the speed of braking down of the starch is dependent of how fast is the amylase activities.

3. **Betaine:** It has significant role in assisting to maintain the balance of vital cell fluid as in Osmolytes

4. **Bromelain:** It makes the meat more tender and serves as an anti-inflammatory agent

Starch is very important component in out diet. Wheat, potatoes, rice, corn, and other staple grains contain the high amount of starch. It almost contains 60% of calories that we intake.

A study was conducted to measure the functional capabilities of the salivary enzymes. Saliva samples from around 50 individuals were taken for research purpose and all of them were adults. Each individual was given a corn starch liquid solution to drink and after the time span of two hour the sample of blood was taken to analyze the blood glucose level. Findings suggested that adults with high amylase activity have found less glucose in their blood. Researchers have confirmed that people with high activities of glucose have more stable level of glucose in their blood.

The saliva has a huge content of enzymes as mentioned earlier and all these enzymes individually and also in group helps the oral system of the body greatly. There are a list of benefits that saliva and its enzyme content has and has been mentioned below in detail.

Makes Speech And Eat Easy

Saliva is 99% water and 1% has all the soluble enzymes and it acts as a lubricant while we eat and while we speak. If someone has a deficiency of this kind of enzymes then he will face trouble in talking and gulping down the food. The saliva in mouth basically contains mucins, which forms the lining of the cell in the mouth. This lining is basically very important for the functions performed by mouth like eating, speaking, brushing and even drinking water.

Making Sensation Possible

We eat food and when we break down the food into various taste they give then we find that some are sweet some are sour. We find that they are spicy, cold and hot and they give out many kinds of sensation to our mouth. Now all these are kind of sensations that our tongue feel while it taste any kind of food. Saliva makes us feel these sensations and if saliva secretion is decreased then we will not feel any kind of sensation. There are taste buds into on top of our tongue and they help us in differentiating between various kinds of taste like sweet and sour and such. This process is also supported by the saliva secretion inside our mouth.

Formation Of Bolus

Bolus is basically the round mass of food particles that we intake. When we take a bite of food then we chew it and while chewing it mixes with the saliva content of mouth and forms a round mass, which is known as bolus. This bolus can be gulped down further. Without the formation of bolus we will not be able to take the food into our digestive system, in its original form. The food that we swallow also has some water in it so the mucin in the saliva also soaks all the water and thus we do not lose any kind of fluid in this process.

Protect From Noxious Substance

When we intake some substances that is not healthy for our mouth lining cells, we are protected by the harmful effects of the substance as the mucins present in saliva helps in protecting the epithelial surface of our mouth, which is nothing but the mouth lining of our mouth. When someone has some kind of dental plague then our mouth starts secreting bad and foul enzymes known as proteolytic enzymes. Mucins present in saliva also save our epithelial surface from these bad enzymes.

Protects The Stomach Lining

The mucins also shield the stomach lining of the body. Inside our stomach there is lot of acid secretion that takes place. This acid is very important for the digestion of the food however; sometimes it also affects the stomach lining badly because of no food being present for the acid to digest. The mucins save the stomach lining from being affected by the acids and if this protective system is not present then our stomach will be damaged seriously. The digestive enzyme, pepsin, that is secreted into the stomach acts regularly on the food we intake and if there is a mismatch between the food taken and the acid secretion then it leads to problem of gas within our stomach. Mucins save our stomach lining from this problem.

Buffering The Acid Generation

The bicarbonate ions those are present in the saliva helps in diluting the acid that is generated from the dietary sugars. It also dilutes the acid generation and thus decreases the harmful effects of the acid. The bicarbonates properties are different from mouth to mouth and also depend upon the time of the day.

Saliva Fights The Micro- Organisms

There are many chemical weapons present in the saliva. These chemical agents are as simple in nature like urea and are as complex in nature like complex proteins. Now our mouth also has micro organisms which are produced into the mouth because of our dietary habits, our health conditions and also because of any health medication that we take. All these micro organisms harm our mouth lining and thus saliva, with the help of its chemical properties, saves our mouth from all such micro organisms. A normal mouth condition is maintained with the help of saliva and its contents. Urea, a content of saliva, is said to have anti- bacterial substances which are also incorporated into tooth pastes that helps in fighting the bacteria of mouth.

Helps In Decreasing Various Bacterial Function In Mouth

There are various bacterial functions which are reduced with the help of saliva and are mentioned below.

- It saves the cellular destruction by destabilizing the cells walls of bacteria.

- It deposits or in words aggregates the cells of bacteria to the point where the functioning of these bacteria is hampered and they cannot damage the soft tissues of mouth.

- Oral flora is also controlled by a chemical present in the saliva known as immune globulin.

Helps In Proper Secretion Of Mouth Glands

The salivary glands are an important part of the mouth as they maintain a proper flow of saliva into our mouth. The proper flow of saliva into mouth ensures that other glands of mouth secrete the substances properly and on a regular flow. This proper secretion ensures that our mouth remain any infection free and functions properly. It also ensures that the there are no calcification s happens with in the ducts in the mouth.

Helps Overcoming Caries

Caries is that state of mouth wherein there is a mismatch between the demineralization and remineralization from the enamel surface of mouth. When we eat something like sugar then the acid produced out of it demineralize the enamel surface of our mouth and it takes time to again revive back and get the mineral ions back into the mouth. This mismatch results in affecting the oral structure of the mouth. Now, if the mouth has a proper secretion of saliva into our mouth then this process of caries does not happen often and thus maintains a proper functioning of our oral structure.

Protects Teeth From Erosive Effects

When we drink erosive drinks, which have acidic effects in them, then it disturbs the teeth. These drinks could be soft drinks those are commonly consumes these days. When we intake these sugar coated acidic drinks then it gets mixed with the saliva in mouth and thus dilutes the acidic content of the drink and then neutralizes the whole content which helps in saving the teeth and getting an erosive effect on the teeth. It also saves the stomach lining from the gastrula affects in the stomach lining.

Saliva Enzyme Production

Apart from the abnormal disease like Sjorgen's syndrome, our mouth is much capable of producing the saliva on its own. It does not take a huge process for proper secretion of the saliva into mouth. Merely by proper chewing of the food, the saliva is secreted properly into our mouth. There are though some kinds of food which secretes the saliva in more content as compared to other food but still proper chewing of the food ensures that the saliva is secreted properly. Lemon juice is one substance which ensures that there is huge secretion of saliva from our salivary glands. The main reason for a decrease in the secretion from our salivary glands is the medication that we take. With age, our medication for various ailments increases and thus with age the secretion from salivary glands decreases and per say, age itself is not a factor for the slow functioning of salivary glands.

Start Of Breakdown Of Food

Mouth is the place where first interaction between the food we intake and our digestive system, takes place. The minor breakdown or the initial breakdown of food happens at mouth. Amylase that is present in the saliva helps in breakdown of carbohydrates that we intake on a regular basis. One will be amazed to know the fact that on a daily basis around 2 liters of saliva is secreted into our body.

Insulation Agent

The saliva content of the mouth helps in proper insulation of the mouth, gums, lips, tongue and the side walls of the mouth. It constantly keeps all the parts of our mouth wet and thus insulates them. Insulation is the process wherein intervention of a substance, making a particular area wet, and thus reduces the release of heat energy from that surface. Now in here the substance that is the wetting agent is saliva and the surface is side walls of mouth, gums, and teeth and thus mentioned earlier.

Natural Substitute Of Water

Saliva acts as a natural water substitute as when we feel some thirst then we gulp down some saliva into our throat. This however, is not a permanent solution for our thirst and one must take proper water when we feel thirsty. When our thirst grows to a higher level then we start feeling dizzy and even intake of saliva does not help our mouth. This is the indication that our body is getting dehydrated and we must take water.

Ejecting Germs

Saliva is 90% water and it collects out all the harmful germs and chemicals present in our mouth and once all these germs and chemicals are collected then we can spit out all the germs along with saliva present in our mouth.

Testing Agent

Just by testing the saliva of our mouth we can determine the body condition. Someone has taken some drug or any kind of chemicals then just by taking a saliva test it can be reveled that whether the person has taken some hard drink or some drugs. Even if we are suffering from some grave disease like cancer or some hormonal imbalance then even that can be detected from the saliva sample of our mouth.

Development Of Taste Buds

Our tongue is considered to be the combination of many taste buds that helps in feeling various kinds of taste and flavors. There are foods which provide various kinds of taste like spicy, sweet, sour, salty, and pungent and many kinds of such taste. All these taste can be actually felt and experienced only because of presence of taste buds and their active working. Saliva is supposed to secrete a hormone known as gustin which actually develops the taste buds. Now, if a person's specific taste is not developed properly then it means that the particular taste bud for that particular component is not developed.

Proper Taste Development

When a person complains of metallic taste in food then it is actually not a problem of food rather it the low level of saliva into the mouth which does not give a proper sense of taste to the person. Saliva is the main substance that ensures that we get a proper sense of taste from the food that we intake. It is through this liquid medium and the chemicals present in it which carries the food to taste receptors cell and a person feels the actual taste of food. If the saliva secretion of the system is not strong then we will actually not be able to feel any kind of taste and get a metallic taste in whatever we eat.

Saliva Enzyme Helping In Wound Cleaning

If a person is hurt and gets a normal cut or wound then he can actually lick that particular wound or cut and can clean off all the pathogens that circulate around that wound. The enzymes resent in saliva helps in the same. Water is no doubt the best medium to clean off all the wounds but if water is in accessible then even saliva can substitute water and can clean off the damaged area. In some species, licking wound with saliva has shown positive results and it has some healing effects on the wound. Saliva contains an enzyme known as NGF which is supposed to have a positive effect in healing the wounds. This substance is also found in saliva of human but because of presence of various other chemicals, saliva does not heal the wounds nevertheless it does help in cleaning them.

Washing Away Sticky Food

We take all kinds of food, raw, cooked and over cooked. Some kinds of food like noodles which has a wax coating on them and also some chocolates that has caramel content in them sticks around our gums and teeth and they decay into our mouth which damages the oral system of our body. These sticky foods are removed away from the corners of our teeth and gums with the help of saliva. When we direct a gush of saliva into the area where the food is stuck it helps in dissolving of such food item and thus helps in removal of the same from our mouth.

Avoiding Parotitis

The enzymes present in the saliva helps in saving the salivary glands from getting infected. The common infection that happens in our glands is known as parotitis, wherein the glands have to suffer inflammation. Inflammation is the medical condition wherein a particular body parts reddens, becomes hot and it becomes painful. The salivary glands are present in both the sides of the mouth and during Parotitis, one or both the glands might be affected. The enzyme content ensures that a person does not have to suffer from this kind of medical condition.

Salivary Enzymes Help In Fats Digestion

The salivary glands present in both sides of our mouth ensure that the proper digestion of fats takes place in the body. Salivary glands secrete an enzyme known as salivary lipase, this particular substance help in digestion of fats. When we intake any food then the enzymes present in saliva actually breaks down the food which is then passed onto the intestine for further break down of food into smallest particles. In infants the pancreatic lipase is not developed properly and it takes time for its development. Till the system is properly ready the infant basically depends upon the salivary lipase for the breakdown of fatty food.

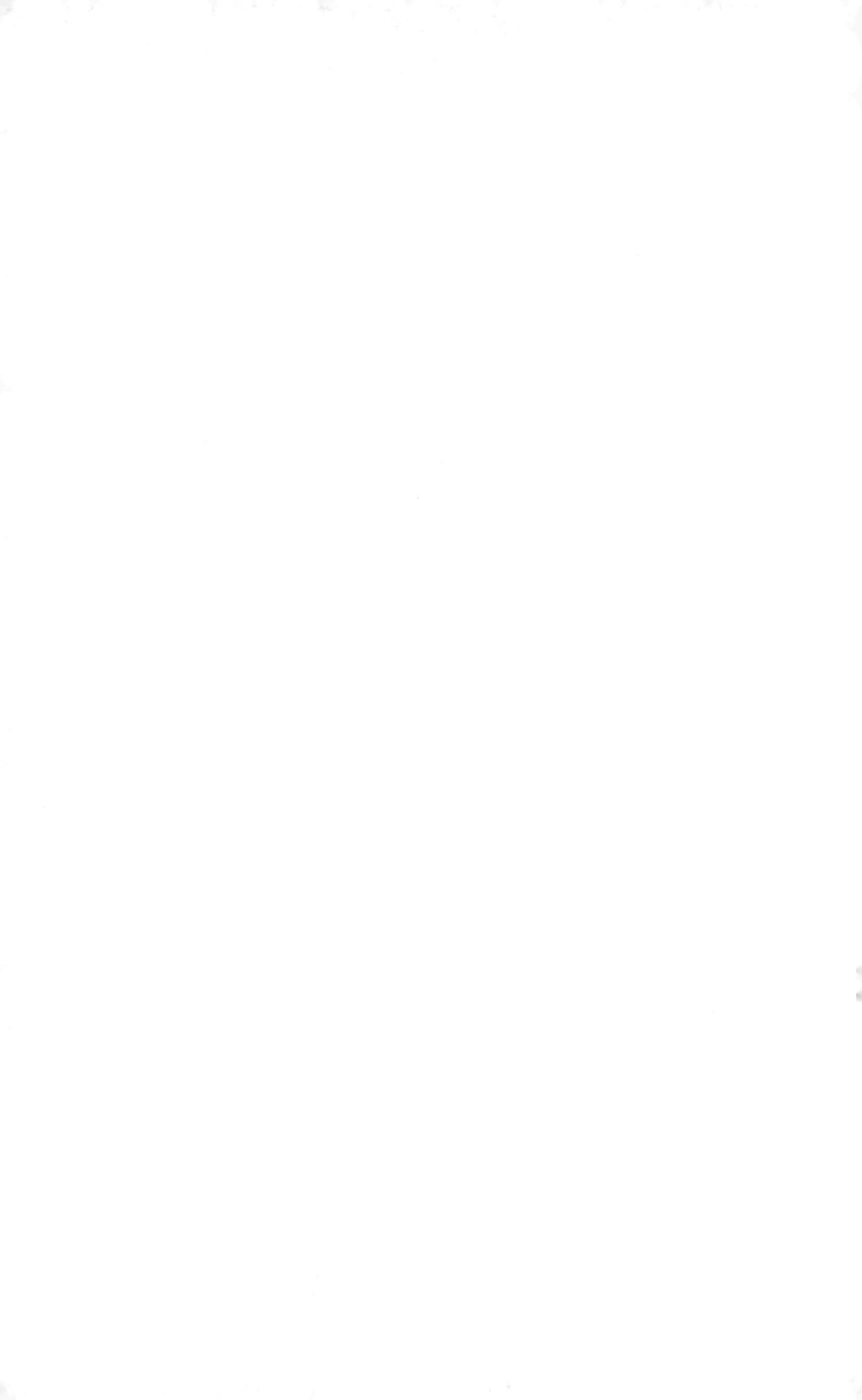

www.ingramcontent.com/pod-product-compliance
Lightning Source LLC
Chambersburg PA
CBHW072014280526
45788CB00005B/2044